Embracing a Vibrant Life with Lichen Sclerosis

The Super Easy Cookbook to Manage Symptoms, Avoid Triggers, Support Immunity, Balance Hormones, and Improve Overall Health

DR LANA BROWN, RN

Copyright Page

© 2024 by Dr. Lana Brown.

For permissions requests, write to the author at www.thelanabrown.com

Table of Contents

CHAPTER I

UNDERSTANDING LICHEN SCLEROSIS

Lichen sclerosis is a disease that attacks the skin. It is an inflammatory health condition that can cause irritable skin changes that comes with pain, discoloration, and itching. It causes a thin-like white patch on the skin, and the affected areas can tear easily. These patches can be present on different parts of a person's body but are commonly found around the anus, vulva, or on the foreskin of the penis. It can also cause sores and blisters to form around the genitals.

Although the primary cause of lichen sclerosis has not been established, healthcare experts believe it is a kind of autoimmune disease because it behaves the same way. Even though it mainly affects women past menopause, it can occur at any age. When left untreated, this inflammatory disease can cause scarring making it extremely painful to have intercourse, urinate, or pass bowels. The symptoms of lichen sclerosis vary; they could be severe or mild. When the disease is mild, one might not experience any symptoms, but the symptoms are bound to manifest when severe.

Lichen sclerosis is a chronic long-term condition that tends to go through cycles where symptoms flare up, then calm down. Without treatment, it can lead to scarring, making it difficult or painful to have sexual intercourse (dyspareunia), urinate (pee) or have a bowel movement (poop). Untreated lichen sclerosis can also increase your chances of developing a type of skin cancer (penile cancer and vulvar squamous cell carcinoma). There isn't a cure for lichen sclerosis, though treatment can help manage your symptoms.

Other names for lichen sclerosis include balanitis xerotica obliterans (BXO) and white spot disease.

What does lichen sclerosis look like?

When lichen sclerosis first appears, it looks like small, white, shiny, slightly raised spots on your genitals or anus. Over time, more spots may develop and eventually join together to form a white patch that looks like wrinkly parchment or tissue paper.

How common is lichen sclerosis?

Lichen sclerosis isn't common. About 200,000 people in the United States have it.

Even if you have several risk factors, lichen sclerosis is still rare.

Symptoms and Diagnosis

Mild cases usually start as shiny white spots on the skin of the vulva in women or on the foreskin of uncircumcised men. It also sometimes affects the area around the anus. In women, it can appear on other body parts—particularly the upper torso, breasts, and arms—but this is rare.

If the disease worsens, itching is the most common symptom, which in rare cases can be extreme enough to interfere with sleep and daily activities. Rubbing or scratching to relieve the itching can cause:

Bleeding

Tearing

Painful sores

Blisters

Bruising

It's a good idea to avoid having sex, wearing tight clothing or tampons, riding a bike, or any other activity that might cause pressure or friction on the affected areas while you are experiencing symptoms. Any trauma, including friction, can cause fragile skin to be damaged and lead to scarring.

Severe Symptoms

In severe cases in women, lichen sclerosis can lead to scarring that causes the inner lips of the vulva to shrink and disappear, the clitoris to become covered with scar tissue, and the opening of the vagina to narrow. People with lichen sclerosis can sometimes experience sexual dysfunction because of these symptoms.

In men with severe lichen sclerosis, the foreskin can scar, tighten, and shrink over the head of the penis, making it hard to pull back the foreskin and decreasing sensation in the tip of the penis. Occasionally, erections are painful, and the urethra (the tube through which urine flows) can become narrow or obstructed, leading to burning or pain during urination and even bleeding during intercourse.

When lichen sclerosis develops around the anus, the discomfort can lead to constipation. This is particularly common in children.

Diagnosis

Anyone who develops symptoms of lichen sclerosis should see a doctor as soon as possible.

Early diagnosis of lichen sclerosis means that treatment can begin immediately. Prompt treatment can prevent the condition from worsening and make it more manageable.

A doctor will often be able to make a diagnosis by carrying out a physical examination of the affected areas. They may want to examine a small sample of skin under a microscope to ensure that the condition is lichen sclerosis.

Occasionally, lichen sclerosis may have no symptoms. When this is the case, a doctor may only diagnose the condition when they are examining the affected area for another unrelated reason.

Causes and Risk Factors

Causes

The cause of lichen sclerosis is unknown, although an overactive immune system may play a role. Some scientists believe that an infectious bacterium called a spirochete may cause changes in the immune system that lead to lichen sclerosis.

Researchers still need to gain an understanding of what can cause a flare-up of lichen sclerosis. However, it is correlated with:

- Hormonal status in women, specifically low levels of estrogen
- Frequent trauma to the skin, including friction
- Autoimmune responses in the body
- Genetic predisposition

It's also possible that certain people have a genetic tendency toward the disease, and studies suggest that abnormal hormone levels may also play a role. Here's what it's helpful to know about this relatively uncommon skin disease that is rarely serious.

Risk Factors

It can affect anyone. But postmenopausal people assigned female at birth (AFAB) between the ages of 40 and 60 are more likely to develop it. People AFAB who haven't gone through puberty also have a higher risk.

Less commonly, lichen sclerosis affects people assigned male at birth (AMAB) who still have their foreskin. You may also have a slightly increased risk if you have an autoimmune disease or allergies.

Diabetes and a body mass index (BMI) greater than 30 (having overweight/obesity) may also increase your risk for lichen sclerosis.

Complications

Serious complications of lichen sclerosis can happen, especially if you don't get treated.

Your skin becomes fragile and can easily be damaged, with bleeding, tears, and open sores that may get infected.

Lichen sclerosis can cause serious scarring to the outer part of the female genitals, called the vulva, and change the way your genitals look and feel.

You may end up with chronic, or ongoing, pain in the vulva and a narrowing of the vaginal opening. These complications can make sex difficult and painful.

If your penis is affected, it can make your foreskin thick and less flexible. You may have a hard time retracting it to clean or to pee (phimosis), or your foreskin could get stuck behind the head of your penis (paraphimosis). You may also have pain during sex and trouble peeing.

You may also be more likely to develop a type of skin cancer on your vulva or penis.

Treatment Approaches

Currently, there is no known cure for lichen sclerosis. However, there are many effective ways to relieve and manage symptoms to ease and minimise discomfort.

Lichen sclerosis can sometimes clear up on its own. This usually happens when it is on parts of the body other than the genital and anal areas.

There are many ways to treat lichen sclerosis around the genital areas, however. Some of these methods are outlined here, but there may be other more recent treatments available. As a result, it is important to discuss treatment options with a doctor.

Corticosteroids

Topical corticosteroids are usually the first line of defense against lichen sclerosis to cure the disease and restore the skin's normal texture and strength.

However, steroids won't reverse any scarring that may have already occurred. And because they're very strong, it's important to contact a healthcare provider frequently to check the skin for side effects when the medication is used daily.

Once symptoms are gone and the skin has regained its strength, the medication can be used less frequently but may still be needed a few times a week to keep lichen sclerosis in remission.

Immune Modulating Medication

If the disease doesn't clear up after a few months of using a topical steroid cream or ointment, a healthcare provider may move on to prescribing a medication that modulates the immune system, such as Protopic (tacrolimus) or Elidel (pimecrolimus). For people who can't tolerate other medications, retinoids may be helpful. Sometimes, too, other factors, such as low estrogen levels that cause vaginal dryness and soreness, a skin infection, or irritation or allergy to the medication, can keep symptoms from clearing up.

Lichen Sclerosis Surgery

Surgery to treat lichen sclerosis that's on your penis can be a good option. Doctors often do a circumcision, which is removing the foreskin--the tissue that covers the head of the penis. After that, the condition probably won't come back.

If you have severe scarring of your vulva that causes problems with sex, surgery can help. But it's only an option once the condition is under control.

Lichen Sclerosis Self-Help

It may be hard, but try not to scratch. That can cause even more damage to fragile skin.

You may be able to soothe the itch by taking baths in a few inches of plain, lukewarm water. Use only a mild cleanser.

Gently pat yourself dry and apply a water-blocking ointment like petroleum jelly to the affected skin. Do the same after you pee so urine doesn't stay on your skin.

Avoid tight clothing, perfumed genital sprays, harsh skin cleansers, and scented dryer or fabric sheets. Don't sit around in wet or sweaty clothing after a swim or a workout.

It may also help to wear cotton underwear during the day and no underwear when sleeping at night.

CHAPTER II

IMPORTANCE OF DIET IN MANAGING LICHEN SCLEROSIS

Although diet is not a cure for lichen sclerosis, it can significantly alleviate the inflammatory condition. A diet containing foods that are low in oxalates can provide benefits that can help reduce pain. This is because high amounts of oxalates in the urine can cause irritation and burn in the vulva. In addition, a study has shown that foods that contain high amounts of oxalates should be avoided when treating lichen sclerosis.

Role of Nutrition in Skin Health

Nutritional status plays an important role in the maintenance of healthy skin. Macronutrients (carbohydrates, proteins, and lipids) and micronutrients (vitamins and nutritionally essential minerals) work together to maintain the barrier functions of skin in the face of everyday challenges. Changes in nutritional status that alter skin structure and function can also directly affect skin appearance. Unlike many organs, skin nutrition may be enhanced directly through topical applications. Topical application of micronutrients can complement dietary consumption, leading to a stronger, healthier protective barrier for the body.

Much of the role of nutrition in skin health focuses on the effects of deficiency, since the structural components of the skin are supported by a variety of nutritive factors, such as small peptides, minerals, and vitamins, which serve as enzyme cofactors, activators, or inhibitors. The skin is also constantly exposed to high concentrations of oxygen, UV light, and oxidizing chemicals, highlighting a role for antioxidant vitamins in skin function. Further, nutritional support of the skin is important for inflammatory response during wound healing.

Common Dietary Triggers and Aggravators

There is little-to-no research on the impact of diet on lichen sclerosis. The Vulval Pain Society provides some research pointing to the potential benefit of diet changes, like a low-oxalate diet, that may affect pain level. Findings are not conclusive, and a low-oxalate diet has been refuted by another study.

This lack of ironclad evidence doesn't mean you should not try a low-oxalate diet, especially if a urine test indicates you have high levels of oxalate in your urine.

Oxalate is a byproduct of your body's metabolism. It's produced naturally by the body and is also found in many plants. High-oxalate foods can cause inflammation in the body's tissues. Oxalate is eliminated from the body through urine and stool.

Reducing the amount of oxalate which passes through your system may help to reduce inflammation from occurring around the vulva and anal region. Eating low-oxalate foods may help, especially when coupled with a calcium citrate supplement, or with high-calcium foods. Calcium binds to oxalate, reducing its absorption into the body's tissues.

CHAPTER III

GENERAL DIETARY GUIDELINES

Beyond being careful about the amount of oxalates you're eating, the following diet tips may help manage symptoms of lichen sclerosis.

1. Consider Adopting an Autoimmune Protocol Diet

Although there are no direct recommendations for a lichen sclerosis diet, there is a strong link to autoimmune disorders, hormone imbalances and autoantibodies, so a diet used to control autoimmune disorders could potentially help with symptoms.

The November 2017 issue of Inflammatory Bowel Diseases describes the autoimmune protocol diet as consisting of a six-week elimination phase during which grains, legumes, nightshades, dairy, eggs, coffee, alcohol, nuts and seeds, refined/processed sugars, oils and food additives are removed from the diet.

This diet is maintained for several weeks and sometimes foods are slowly reintroduced to observe if symptoms return. This can help target offending foods. In other cases, people with autoimmune diseases may choose to keep these foods out of the diet indefinitely.

This type of elimination diet can be tricky to do on your own, so it's a good idea to enlist the help of your doctor or a dietitian, to make sure you're still getting the nutrients you need.

2. Add a Calcium Citrate Supplement

As we noted above, calcium binds to oxalates in your body. If you don't get enough high-calcium foods in your diet, you may want to take a calcium supplement. Calcium citrate is the preferred form, according to the Cleveland Clinic.

3. Drink Plenty of Water

Make sure to drink plenty of H_2O throughout the day, which will help you stay hydrated but also thin out your urine, which can prevent the buildup of chemicals that can irritate lichen sclerosis. The Cleveland Clinic recommends drinking 10 to 12 cups of fluid daily, with at least five of those cups being water.

Foods to Include for a Lichen Sclerosis-friendly diet

1. Omega-3 fatty acids

These acids can help regulate the rate at which the skin produces oil, enhance hydration, suppress breakouts, and minimize the signs of aging. Consuming foods that contain omega-3 fatty acids in your lichen sclerosis diet can help reduce the roughness of skin patches by providing a soothing effect to the irritated area. In a small study, women who consumed flaxseed oil, which is rich in omega-3 fatty acids, for twelve weeks, developed less sensitive and rough skin. Incorporating foods that contain generous amounts of omega-3 fatty acids can help boost skin barriers, thereby preventing skin conditions. Moreover, foods with omega-3 fatty acids reduce the risk of skin cancer, enhance wound healing, and decrease hair loss. Foods that contain omega-3 fatty acids include soybean oil, cold chia seeds, tuna, walnuts, and canola oil.

2. Vegetables

A great source of powerful vitamins and nutrients, vegetables can help strengthen the immune system, thereby preventing the onset of disease. Consuming vegetables can also reduce the symptoms of lichen sclerosis, but it is vital to ensure that you are only consuming vegetables that are low in oxalates. They include radishes, water chestnuts, zucchini, Brussels sprouts, chives, cabbage, endive, cucumbers, and mushrooms. In addition, vegetables can help improve mental health, boost heart health, enhance the health of the gut and digestive system, and prevent chronic diseases.

3. Cooked and dry cereals

Cereals are loaded with complex carbohydrates to prevent constipation, improve energy levels, and reduce high blood sugars. Cereal grains can also improve your health by providing the body with beneficial minerals, fats, vitamins, proteins, and lipids. When eating for lichen sclerosis, it is important to opt for dry and cooked cereals that contain little or no oxalates. Some examples include Cheerios, Rice Krispies, and Rice Chex. However, because these kinds of cereals are made from refined grains, try to refrain from eating them consistently and make sure you consume them with fruits to obtain all the necessary ingredients that your body needs. In addition, ensure the cereals do not contain bran or nuts.

4. Parmesan cheese

Also referred to as 'Parmigiano Reggiano', Parmesan cheese is an Italian cheese with nutritional contents that can decrease the risk of certain diseases. Parmesan cheese has high amounts of calcium and protein, and a one-ounce serving of Parmesan cheese contains up to 26% of the daily calcium our bodies require. According to studies, calcium can help reduce the number of oxalates the body absorbs. Other health advantages that you can get from consuming Parmesan cheese include enhanced bone health and better absorption of minerals like zinc and iron. Moreover, Parmesan cheese contains important amino acids that the body needs. Our body requires these amino acids to perform essential processes like the developing hormones and body tissue repair.

5. Fruits

Fruits containing a tiny amount of oxalates or none include cherries, bananas, yellow plums, nectarines, green plums, grapefruit, mangoes, and melons. A diet rich in fruits can reduce the risk of developing several diseases such as cancer, inflammatory disease, and diabetes. Fruits like bananas contain an amazing amount of potassium that can aid the reduction of anxiety, and high blood pressure and prevent strokes. Fruits are beneficial in helping to upgrade the functions of the immune system.

Watermelons, apples, and grapes are examples of some fruits that you consume for an enhanced immune system.

In summary, Low-oxalate foods and drinks include:

• poultry

• fish

• beef

• dairy products, such as cow's milk, goat's milk, and cheese

• avocados

• apples

• melon

• grapes

• peaches

• plums

• broccoli

• asparagus

• cauliflower

• lettuce

• white chocolate

• green peas

• all oils, including olive oil, and vegetable oil

• herbs, and seasonings, such as salt, white pepper, basil, and cilantro

• beer, and most forms of alcohol

• coffee

• weak, lightly-steeped green tea

Foods to Avoid or Limit

It is recommended to avoid the following foods, as they can enhance the symptoms of the disease and make the pain more severe. They are high in oxalates which can cause skin irritability and burning sensations. In addition, make sure you stay away from foods that can increase inflammation.

Here is a list of lichen sclerosis foods to avoid:

Okra

Rhubarb

Spinach

Soybeans

Miso soup

Corn grits

Raspberries

Bulgur

Beets

French fries

Processed meat, such as sausage and hot dog

Bagels

Almonds

Margarine and lard

Tobacco

Alcohol

Lentil soup

Brown rice flour

Bran flakes

All forms of potatoes — whether baked or fried

CHAPTER IV

NUTRIENTS AND SUPPLEMENTS

Your skin needs the right balance of nutrients to do its main job: a barrier that protects the rest of your body from things outside it. To help keep your skin looking, working, and feeling good, feed it well from the inside.

Healthy Fats

This is how your skin gets its "glow." Too little fat in your diet can make your skin wrinkled and dry.

Focus on monounsaturated and polyunsaturated fats from plants like nuts, seeds, and avocados and from fish. These help your skin stay moist, firm, and flexible, and they're better for your heart than saturated fats.

Omega-3 fatty acids are a kind of polyunsaturated fat, which your body can't make but needs to build cell walls. They also block a chemical that lets skin cancer grow and spread, and they may lower inflammation.

Protein

Your body turns the proteins you eat into building blocks called amino acids and reuses them to make other proteins, including the collagen and keratin that form the structure of skin. Amino acids also help slough off old skin.

Some amino acids are antioxidants that protect skin cells against UV rays and from "free radicals" made when your body breaks down certain foods or is around cigarette smoke.

Vitamin A

Both the upper and lower layers of skin need vitamin A. It seems to prevent sun damage by interrupting the process that breaks down collagen. Since it's an antioxidant, it may give your skin some protection against sunburn (although not as much as wearing sunscreen). It helps the oil glands around your hair follicles work and may also help cuts and scrapes heal, especially if you're taking steroids to reduce inflammation.

Without enough vitamin A, your skin might get dry and itchy or bumpy.

Vitamin C

Think "C" for collagen: This vitamin helps the twisted web of protein hold its shape. It's also a powerful antioxidant, protecting you from free radicals and possibly lowering your chance of skin cancer. Low levels of vitamin C can cause easy bruising and bleeding gums, as well as slower-healing sores.

Vitamin E

This antioxidant and anti-inflammatory can also absorb the energy from UV light, which damages skin and leads to wrinkles, sagging, and skin cancer. It works with vitamin C to strengthen cell walls.

Zinc

The outer layer of your skin has five times more of this mineral than the layer underneath. Zinc helps your skin heal after an injury. It's needed to keep cell walls stable and for cells to divide and specialize as they grow.

Zinc may protect skin from UV damage because of the way it behaves in relation to other metals in your body, like iron and copper. It also acts like an antioxidant.

Too little zinc can look like eczema, but the itchy rash won't get better when you put moisturizers and steroid creams on it.

Selenium

Selenium is a mineral that helps certain antioxidants protect your skin from UV rays. Selenium deficiency has been linked with a greater chance of skin cancer.

Foods and Supplements

In general, fruits and vegetables are good choices because they have skin-friendly vitamins and other antioxidants.

Some foods pack more than one nutrient for your skin, which often helps them work better:

• Fatty fish (salmon, sardines, tuna): protein, omega-3s, selenium

• Leafy dark greens (kale, spinach, collards): vitamins A, C, and E; omega-3s; protein plus selenium in spinach

• Eggs: protein, vitamins A and E, selenium, zinc

• Flaxseeds: omega-3s, selenium

• Legumes (lentils, chickpeas): protein, zinc

• Avocados: healthy fats, vitamins C and E

• Extra virgin olive oil: healthy fats, vitamin E

Talk to your doctor if you're concerned you're not getting enough of these key nutrients from your food to make sure supplements won't affect your health in other ways. Fish oil is a source of omega-3s, for example, but taking it may not be a good idea if you're on blood thinners or have a weakened immune system. And zinc supplements can make some antibiotics less effective.

Recommended Supplements for Lichen Sclerosis

Some supplements that may help lichen sclerosis are:

• L-glutamine, aloe, and slippery elm, which can support gut health and reduce inflammation.

• Liquid fish oil, B group vitamins, and zinc, which can reduce inflammation and fight infection.

• Calendula, chickweed, and gotu kola, which are herbs that have anti-inflammatory, antifungal, and antibacterial properties and may improve healing of lesions.

• Curcumin and quercetin, which are natural anti-inflammatories that may address immune response.

• Apple cider vinegar, castor oil, lavender oil, aloe vera, borax, baking soda, emu oil, and coconut oil, which are home remedies that may reduce dryness, irritation, swelling, and infection.

Herbal Remedies and their Benefits

For those looking for a natural approach, these herbs or a combination of them can be used at the first sign of skin irritation.

Comfrey- (Symphytum officinale) is used for it's tissue healing benefits. Comfrey, also known as knit bone, helps to "knit" the damaged cells back together. Comfrey helps heals wounds in short time. The wounded area must be clean, as comfrey works fast. If the area is dirty, infection can start as the germs are trapped inside. Comfrey is an emoillent herb, and helps to form a protective layer so skin can heal.

Calendula (Calendula officinalis) is the best herb to have for skin conditions. It is antibacterial, anti-fungal, and antiseptic. It's wound healing properties helps to fight skin infections.

Chickweed (Stellaria media) helps to reduce the itch that is associated with Lichen Sclerosis. Chickweed helps to stop the itch in just minutes.

Lavender (Lavendula Angustifolia) Wound healer. Lavender helps to heal wounds safely. Lavender acts as an anti-bacterial, and antiseptic agent.

Red Clover (Trifolium pratense) is used as a topical anti-inflammatory. It helps heal wounds, and has some phyto estrogen effects. This has been shown to help heal lichen in menopausal women.

Plantain (Plantago major) is a wonderful herb to help stop the itch on skin. It's chemical herbal properties stop the itch of lichen if used regularly.

Witch Hazel-(Hamamelis virginian) is an astringent, and will help dry the skin, without over drying. It also acts as a protection against getting infections. This is the herb, and not the witch hazel you buy in the drug store.

CHAPTER V

NOURISHING BREAKFAST RECIPES FOR LICHEN SCLEROSIS

2 Ingredient English Muffin Recipe

INGREDIENTS

• 2 teaspoon butter

• 1½ cups mozzarella cheese shredded

• 2 large eggs

INSTRUCTIONS

1. Preheat the oven to 350 °F (175°C). Grease a 6-cup muffin pan with butter.

2. Combine cheese and eggs together in a large mixing bowl.

3. Divide the batter and fill each muffin space evenly.

4. Bake for 20 minutes, until tops are golden brown.

5. Run a knife around the edges to loosen each muffin. Remove from the pan and cool on a wire rack.

Hot Keto Cereal (Low-Carb Oatmeal)

INGREDIENTS

- ½ cup coconut flour

- ¼ cup flax seed

- ¼ cup chia seed

- 3 cups water

- ¼ cup Keto sugar substitute

- 1 teaspoon ground cinnamon

- 1 teaspoon vanilla extract

- ¼ teaspoon salt

- 4 whole eggs whisked

- 4 tablespoons coconut cream

Optional Add-ins:

- ¼ cup berries

- 1 tablespoon almond butter

- 1 tablespoon unsweetened shredded coconut

- 1 tablespoon hemp seeds

- 1 tablespoon cacao nibs

INSTRUCTIONS

1. Combine coconut flour, flax, and chia with the water in a small saucepan over medium heat. Cook for about 5 minutes, as it comes to a simmer.

2. Mix sweeter, cinnamon, vanilla, and salt in a small bowl. Add to the pot and stir to combine.

3. Reduce heat to low. Stir in the whisked eggs and continue cooking until cereal has thickened, approximately 5 minutes.

4. Serve warm with cream on top. Divide optional add-ins equally between all servings.

Carnivore Pancakes Recipe with 2-Ingredients

INGREDIENTS

- 4 ounces cream cheese

- 4 large eggs

- 1 teaspoon butter for frying

Optional Add-ins

- ¼ teaspoon salt

- 1 tablespoon Keto sugar substitute

- ½ tablespoon butter for serving

- ½ cup whipped cream for serving

• 1 tablespoon honey or maple, for serving, if not keto

INSTRUCTIONS

1. Blend the cream cheese and eggs in a blender.

2. Heat the butter in a skillet over medium heat.

3. Scoop the batter with a 1 tablespoon a measuring spoon and pour onto the pan.

4. Cook, until the edges separate from the pan and you can easily slip a spatula under the pancake to flip it over.

5. Flip and cook the second side until it turns golden brown.

6. Remove from heat and set aside. Then, continue cooking all the batter until done.

2-Ingredient Keto Waffles (Flourless Waffles)

INGREDIENTS

• 2 large eggs

• ½ cup shredded cheddar cheese

Optional Toppings

• ½ tablespoon butter

• ¼ cup whipped cream

• ¼ cup raspberries

• 2 tablespoons Sugar-free maple syrup

INSTRUCTIONS

1. Preheat the waffle maker to medium-high heat.

2. Whisk the eggs in a mixing bowl. Mix the cheese until combined.

3. Pour batter into the waffle maker. Close and cook for 3-5 minutes until done. Repeat, if needed, until all batter is cooked.

4. Serve immediately. Store leftovers in the fridge for 3-5 days.

Bone Broth Latte Recipe for Breakfast in the Morning

INGREDIENTS

• ¾ cup freshly brewed coffee hot

• ½ cup bone broth

- ¼ cup milk dairy or plant-based

- 1 ½ tablespoon Keto sugar substitute or sweetener of choice

- 1 tablespoon butter or coconut oil for dairy-free

- 1 raw egg yolk optional

- 1 tablespoon cacao powder

- ½ teaspoon ground cinnamon

- ¼ teaspoon vanilla extract

INSTRUCTIONS

1. Pour the bone broth into a small saucepan and heat it gently over medium-low heat until it becomes hot and steaming but not boiling.

2. Whisk in the sweetener, butter, optional egg yolk, cacao powder, cinnamon, and vanilla until everything blends well.

3. Pour into your favorite mug, and combine with the coffee.

4. Heat the milk in the small saucepan over medium-low heat until it is warm and steaming but not boiling. Froth the milk using a milk frother or by vigorously whisking it by hand in the saucepan until it becomes frothy.

5. Pour the frothed milk over the hot coffee broth. Garnish with an optional dusting of cinnamon. Serve immediately.

The Best Psyllium Husk Keto Bread

INGREDIENTS

• 6 tablespoons psyllium husk powder

• ¾ cup coconut flour

• 1 ½ teaspoons baking soda

• 1 teaspoon salt

• 8 whole eggs

• ½ cup coconut oil or butter, softened

• ¾ cup hot water

INSTRUCTIONS

1. Preheat oven to 350 °F (175°C).

2. Separate the ingredients by mixing the dry ingredients (psyllium husk powder, coconut flour, baking soda, salt) in a bowl and the wet ingredients

(eggs, butter or coconut oil, and hot water) in another bowl.

3. Combine the two bowls together by adding the wet into the dry. Work quickly to mix thoroughly because once the psyllium is activated with water it gels fast! Do not over mix.

4. Transfer to a lightly greased standard 8x4-inch bread loaf pan.

5. Bake for 60 minutes. The best way to tell if the bread is done is to look for a hard and crusty top. It should be dark brown and firm.

6. Remove from the oven and let sit in the bread pan for 15 minutes to settle. Loosen the edges with a knife to release the bread. Cool completely on a wire rack before slicing.

Carnivore Breakfast Muffins (with 5 Keto Variations)

INGREDIENTS

- 9 large eggs

- 8 ounces ground beef

- 1 teaspoon salt

INSTRUCTIONS

1. Preheat the oven to 350 °F (175°C).

2. Lightly grease a standard size muffin tin.

3. Brown the meat in a skillet over medium heat.

4. Whisk eggs in a large bowl. Add meat and salt. Stir to combine.

5. Divide the mixture evenly into the muffin tins. Fill each well ¾ full. Bake for 20 minutes until eggs set.

6. Remove from oven and cool for 5 minutes. Release by running a knife around the edge of each muffin. Pop out and continue cooling on a wire rack or serve. Enjoy leftovers cold or reheat in the oven before serving.

High Protein Strawberry Cheesecake Parfait

INGREDIENTS

• 1/2 cup low-sodium cottage cheese

• 1 tsp vanilla

• 1 tbsp no sugar cheesecake jello pudding (the powder)

• 1/2 cup strawberries

• 1/2 cup non-fat plain Greek yogurt

• 1 tsp honey

INSTRUCTIONS

1. Put all **INGREDIENTS** into mini Cuisinart and blend.

Valentine's Day Protein Packed Parfait

INGREDIENTS

• 4 tart cherries

• 1 tsp vanilla extract

• squirt of lime juice

• 1/2 scoop Vanilla Egg White Protein powder

• 1/2 cup non fat plain Greek yogurt

• 1/2 cup Farmer's Cheese

• mint sprig

• 1/8 cup chopped unsalted Pistachio nuts

INSTRUCTIONS

1. Gather Farmer's cheese, yogurt, protein powder, a squeeze of lime juice, and vanilla and mix in a small Cuisinart or blender.

2. Chop pistachios

3. Put mixed **INGREDIENTS** in a cup and top with cherries, and a tiny bit of lime zest, and chopped pistachios. A sprig of mint will be the surprise hit! Don't skip it!

Copycat Fiber One Muffins

INGREDIENTS

• 1/2 Teaspoon vanilla

• 1 Egg

• 1.5 Cup Fiber One cereal

• 1/2 Cup Swerve brown sugar

• 1/4 Olive oil

• 1 1/3 Cup of Fairlife ultra milk

• Scoop vanilla protein powder

• 1 Cup Bob red mill high fiber oat bran cereal

• 2 teaspoon baking powder

INSTRUCTIONS

1. Preheat oven to 400.

2. Spray the muffin pan with cooking spray so the muffins don't stick.

3. Crush cereal in a baggie with a rolling pin or use a glass like I did. Whatever you have available to crush cereal into a finer consistency.

4. Add milk and vanilla to the cereal and let sit for 5 minutes.

5. In another bowl, beat egg and add in oil.

6. Add the rest of the **INGREDIENTS** (baking powder, protein powder, oat bran, and Swerve brown sugar) to the beaten egg and oil mixture.

7. Add egg mixture to cereal mixture.

8. Fill the muffin pan.

9. Place in oven and bake for 20 minutes. Check at 15 with a toothpick; if it comes out clean, they are done. If not, bake for an additional 5 minutes.

Banana French Toast with Peanut Butter Maple Drizzle

INGREDIENTS

• 1 small banana

- 1 teaspoon cinnamon

- 2 Tablespoon powdered peanut butter

- 1 pat of butter

- Ezekiel bread

- 1/4 cup of skim milk

- 1 whole egg

- 1 Tablespoon sugar-free maple syrup

INSTRUCTIONS

French toast batter.

1. Mix together milk, egg, and cinnamon.

2. Heat a nonstick skillet with a pat of butter.

3. Drench the bread in the batter.

4. When the skillet is hot, put in french toast and cook on each side until brown. About 2 minutes each.

5. While making french toast, make your PB drizzle by following the directions on the PB2 jar. I added more water so that the drizzle could, well, drizzle!

6. When both pieces of toast are nice and brown, put them on the plate and pour on the maple syrup and PB drizzle. Garnish with fruit.

Arugula Egg Goat Cheese Breakfast Wrap

INGREDIENTS

• 1/4 cup tomato, diced

- 1/2 cup arugula

- 1/2 teaspoon coconut oil

- 1 large eggs, beaten

- 1/8 cup goat cheese

- 1 low carb tortilla

INSTRUCTIONS

STEP 1

Warm tortilla in a large skillet over medium heat.

STEP 2

Melt coconut oil in a skillet over medium-high heat.

STEP 3

Add eggs and scramble. Cook for about 2 minutes, sprinkle goat cheese over eggs, add arugula, and continue cooking until cheese is melted.

STEP 4

Add eggs to tortilla and top with diced tomato.

STEP 5

Roll tortilla and enjoy.

Flourless Banana Pancakes

INGREDIENTS

• 1 ripe banana

• 2 large eggs

- 2 tablespoon ground flax meal

- 1/4 teaspoon vanilla

- 1 tablespoon coconut oil

INSTRUCTIONS

1. Mix banana and eggs together in a bowl until smooth. Add ground flaxseed and vanilla extract; mix the batter well.

2. Heat coconut oil in a small skillet over medium-low heat. Scoop batter, about 1/4 cup per pancake, onto the skillet and cook until the center starts to bubble, about 30 seconds. Flip pancakes and cook until bottoms are lightly browned, 1 to 2 minutes more.

Chicken Salad Stuffed Avocado

INGREDIENTS

- 1 tablespoon of cilantro

- 3 ounces chicken (can make own or use rotisserie)

- 3 cherry tomatoes

- 1 tablespoon goat cheese

- 1/2 avocado

INSTRUCTIONS

1. Cut one ripe avocado in half and scoop into bowl. Save the shell as you will use it for serving.

2. Add 3 ounces of cooked chicken (store-bought rotisserie works great!) and mix with avocado.

3. Cut up and mix in three cherry tomatoes.

4. Put mixture back into empty avocado shell.

5. Top it off with goat cheese and cilantro.

CHAPTER VI

NOURISHING LUNCH RECIPES FOR LICHEN SCLEROSIS

Roasted new potato, kale & feta salad with avocado

Ingredients

• 200g Jersey Royal potatoes, halved

• 2 garlic cloves

• 2 tbsp cold-pressed rapeseed oil

• 1 lemon, juiced

• 1 banana shallot, chopped

- 200g bag kale

- 1 small ripe avocado, flesh scooped out

- ½ tsp Dijon mustard

- 25g feta (or vegetarian alternative), crumbled

- ½-1 tsp chilli flakes

- 1 tbsp pumpkin seeds, toasted

Directions

- STEP 1

Heat oven to 200C/180C fan/gas 6. Boil the potatoes for 10 mins until mostly tender, drain and leave to steam dry. Toss the potatoes in a large roasting tin with the garlic, drizzle over 1 tbsp oil and season. Roast for 20 mins.

• STEP 2

While the potatoes are roasting, squeeze half the lemon juice over the shallot and half of the kale, season, then massage gently to encourage the kale to soften.

• STEP 3

Remove the garlic cloves from the oven. Put the rest of the kale on top of the potatoes, drizzle over a little oil, season and return to the oven for 5 mins until crisp.

• STEP 4

Meanwhile, blitz the garlic, avocado, mustard, remaining oil and lemon juice together, add enough water to create a smooth dressing and season to taste. Mix the potatoes and cooked kale into the raw kale salad and tip onto a platter. Drizzle over the dressing, then top with the feta, chilli flakes and pumpkin seeds.

Leek, kale & potato soup topped with shoestring fries

Ingredients

• 4 large potatoes (around 500g), 3 peeled and cubed, 1 left whole with skin on

• 1 tbsp cold pressed rapeseed oil

• 15g butter

• 5 leeks (around 500g), washed and sliced into half moons

• 2 garlic cloves, sliced

• 1 ½l vegetable stock (we used Bouillon)

• 200g kale

• 2 tbsp half-fat crème fraîche

Directions

• STEP 1

Heat oven to 220C/200C fan/ gas 7 and line a baking tray with parchment. Cut the whole potato into matchsticks using a julienne peeler, or shave thin slices using a vegetable peeler, then cut into matchsticks. Pat dry using kitchen paper, then toss with the oil and some seasoning. Spread out on the tray and roast for 15-18 mins.

• STEP 2

Melt the butter in a large saucepan. Add the leeks, chopped potatoes and a pinch of salt, then cook gently for 10 mins until the leeks have softened. Stir in the garlic and cook for 1 min more, then pour in the stock. Simmer for 10-12 mins until the potatoes are soft, then add the kale and cook for 2-3 mins to wilt.

• STEP 3

Stir in the crème fraîche, then blitz with a hand blender and season to taste. Divide the soup between bowls and top with the shoestring fries.

Kale & goat's cheese frittata

Ingredients

• 1 tbsp olive oil

• 2 red onions, thinly sliced

• 200g chopped curly kale

• 2 tbsp balsamic vinegar

• 8 large eggs, lightly beaten with a little seasoning

• 100g firm goat's cheese, broken into chunks

Directions

• STEP 1

Heat oven to 190C/170C fan/gas 5. Heat the oil in a 25cm ovenproof frying pan. Add the onions and cook for 10-15 mins until soft and caramelised. Add the kale and 1 tbsp water, and cook for 5 mins until the kale has wilted. Pour in the balsamic vinegar and bubble for 1 min, then add the eggs. Give everything a quick stir, then leave undisturbed to cook over a low-medium heat for 5 mins until the egg is nearly set and the frittata is turning golden brown on the bottom.

• STEP 2

Scatter the goat's cheese over the top of the frittata. Cook in the oven for 10-15 mins until the cheese is bubbling and the frittata is set in the centre.

Griddled squid, lentil, roast pepper & preserved lemon with tahini

Ingredients

• 3 large red peppers, halved and deseeded

• 4 tbsp extra virgin olive oil, plus a little extra for roasting and frying

- ½ small onion, finely chopped

- 1 celery stick, diced

- 225g puy lentils

- 1 lemon, juiced

- ½ small bunch parsley, chopped

- 600g cleaned and prepared squid

- 2 green and 2 red chillies, halved, deseeded and finely sliced

- 2 garlic cloves, finely sliced

- 1 preserved lemon, flesh removed and discarded, rind very finely sliced

For the tahini dressing

- 4 tbsp tahini

- 2 tbsp Greek yogurt

- 2 tbsp extra virgin olive oil

- 2 garlic cloves, crushed

- ½ lemon, juiced

- ½ small bunch coriander, finely chopped

Directions

- STEP 1

Heat the oven to 200C/180C fan/ gas 6. Put the peppers on a baking tray and brush with some olive oil. Roast for 25-30 mins, until soft and blistered. Leave to cool slightly.

• STEP 2

To make the dressing, combine everything together until it is the consistency of double cream. If it's too thick, add a little water and adjust the seasoning to taste. Set aside. Slice the peppers into strips.

• STEP 3

Heat a little olive oil in a medium pan and fry the onion and celery for 10 mins until soft but not coloured. Tip in the lentils and cover with water. Bring to the boil, then reduce the heat and simmer for 15 mins, or until the lentils are tender, topping up the water if needed.

• STEP 4

Drain the lentils, then spoon into a serving bowl. Season well, then stir in 1 tbsp olive oil, half the lemon juice and the parsley. Leave to cool a bit, then add the peppers.

• STEP 5

Cut the 'wings' from the squid and put them aside with the tentacles. Slice the bodies down one side so they open out, then clean the inside by running a knife blade firmly over the flesh. Score the flesh on the inside, ensuring you don't cut all the way through. Pat dry with kitchen paper, then transfer to a bowl with just enough olive oil to moisten the pieces (about 2 tbsp). Heat a griddle pan until very hot.

• STEP 6

Season the squid and griddle in batches for 20-30 seconds on each side until just golden. Cut into bite-sized pieces, then toss through the lentil salad and drizzle over the remaining lemon juice.

• STEP 7

In a small frying pan, heat 1 tbsp oil and fry the chillies and garlic until golden. Pour over the squid, then toss through the preserved lemon. Serve with the dressing spooned over or on the side.

Sweet & sour radicchio with toasted crumbs & herby lentils

Ingredients

• 5 tbsp extra virgin olive oil or rapeseed oil, plus extra for drizzling

• 1 small red onion, finely chopped

- 15g flat-leaf parsley, leaves picked and finely chopped, stalks finely chopped

- 2 garlic cloves, crushed

- 400g can black or green lentils, drained

- 15g mint, leaves picked and finely chopped

- 3 tbsp sherry or red wine vinegar

- 100g sourdough or focaccia, pulsed to fine crumbs in a food processor

- 1 radicchio (about 500g), quartered, cored and leaves separated

Directions

- STEP 1

Heat 1 tbsp of the oil in a medium saucepan over a medium heat and fry the onion with a pinch of sea salt flakes for 4-5 mins until starting to soften but not colour.

• STEP 2

Add the parsley stalks and half the garlic to the onions, then tip in the lentils and 300ml water. Bring to a simmer and cook for 5 mins, shuffling the pan occasionally – when ready, the lentils should be loose and a little brothy (but not soupy). Add two-thirds of the chopped parsley leaves, two-thirds of the mint, 1 tbsp more oil and 2 tsp of the vinegar. Simmer for 2 mins, then reduce the heat to low just to keep warm.

• STEP 3

Meanwhile, heat 2 tbsp of the oil in a large frying pan over a medium- high heat. After 45 seconds or so, fry the breadcrumbs for 3-4 mins, tossing to coat and stirring occasionally until golden. Reduce the heat to low, stir in the remaining garlic and parsley leaves, cook for 1 min, then transfer to a bowl. Wipe the pan clean with kitchen paper.

• STEP 4

Heat another 1 tbsp oil in the pan over a medium-high heat and cook the radicchio leaves for 1 min, turning often using tongs until they become glossy and slightly wilted (you may need to do this in batches at first, then put all the leaves in the pan once they've all wilted). Make a gap in the middle using a spoon and add the rest of the vinegar along with 1 tbsp water. Turn off the heat and quickly stir the leaves around the pan to wilt further in the steam. Season with sea salt and the remaining mint.

• STEP 5

Divide the lentils between two shallow bowls or plates. Drizzle with a little more oil, top with the leaves and any pan juices, and scatter over the crumbs to serve.

Veggie shepherd's pie with sweet potato mash

Ingredients

• 1 tbsp olive oil

• 1 large onion, halved and sliced

• 2 large carrots (500g/1lb 2oz in total), cut into sugar-cube size pieces

• 2 tbsp thyme chopped

* 200ml red wine

* 400g can chopped tomatoes

* 2 vegetable stock cubes

* 410g can green lentils

* 950g sweet potatoes, peeled and cut into chunks

* 25g butter

* 85g vegetarian mature cheddar, grated

Directions

* STEP 1

Heat 1 tbsp olive oil in a frying pan, then fry 1 halved and sliced large onion until golden.

• STEP 2

Add 2 large carrots, cut into sugar-cube size pieces and most of the 2 tbsp chopped thyme, reserving a sprinkling for later.

• STEP 3

Pour in 200ml red wine, 150ml water and a 400g chopped tomatoes, then crumble in 2 vegetable stock cubes and simmer for 10 mins.

• STEP 4

Tip in a 410g can green lentils, including the juice, then cover and simmer for another 10 mins until the carrots still have a bit of bite and the lentils are pulpy.

• STEP 5

Meanwhile, boil 950g sweet potatoes, cut into chunks, for 15 mins until tender, drain well, then mash with 25g butter and season to taste.

• STEP 6

Pile the lentil mixture into a pie dish, spoon the mash on top, then sprinkle over 85g grated vegetarian mature cheddar and the remaining thyme. The pie can now be covered and chilled for 2 days, or frozen for up to a month.

• STEP 7

Heat oven to 190C/170C fan/gas 5. Cook for 20 mins if cooking straightaway, or for 40 mins from chilled, until golden and hot all the way through. Serve with broccoli.

Lentil & red pepper salad with a soft egg

Ingredients

• 2 eggs

• 400g can green lentils, rinsed and drained

• 1 small red onion, thinly sliced

• 1 red pepper, finely chopped

• 1 tbsp balsamic vinegar

• handful rocket leaves

• 1 tbsp olive oil

Directions

• STEP 1

Boil the eggs for 6 mins, then quickly cool under cold running water and peel off the shells. Tip the lentils into a bowl with the onion, red pepper and balsamic vinegar. Mix well.

• STEP 2

Put the salad onto a serving dish, then pile the rocket on top. Drizzle with the oil, then halve the eggs and sit them on top of the salad.

Salmon meatballs in spicy lentil gravy

Ingredients

• 2 medium slices white bread

• 450g salmon fillet, cut into rough chucks

• 1 egg white

• 1 tbsp olive oil

For the spicy gravy

• 2 tbsp korma curry paste

• 1 small onion, finely chopped

• 2 red peppers, finely chopped

• 500g carton tomato passata

• 50g red lentils

Directions

• STEP 1

In a food processor, whizz the bread to fine crumbs.
Set aside, then whizz the salmon. Add the crumbs
and egg white, then pulse to combine. Season.

Divide into 12 balls and chill for 30 mins. Can be frozen at this stage for up to 1 month.

• STEP 2

Heat oven to 200C/fan 180C/gas 6. Heat the oil in a non-stick frying pan. Add the fishballs and fry for 1-2 mins until lightly browned. Transfer to a baking tray, bake for 15 mins until golden.

• STEP 3

Wipe the pan, add korma paste and onion, and cook for 5 mins, stirring regularly. Add peppers and cook for 2 mins. Add passata and lentils, bring to the boil, then simmer for 20 mins. Coat fishballs in the gravy and serve.

Coriander roast chicken thighs with puy lentil salad

Ingredients

• 185g puy lentils

• 20g ginger, peeled

• 30g coriander, plus extra leaves to serve

• 1 tsp each garam masala and ground coriander

• ½ tsp ground cumin

• 2 large whole garlic cloves, plus 1 small clove, finely grated

• 2 tbsp lemon juice

* 150g pot plain bio yogurt

* 6 bone-in, skinless chicken thighs

* 1 tbsp fresh turmeric, finely grated

* 1 tbsp rapeseed or olive oil, plus 1 tsp

* 3 red onions (325g), thickly sliced

* 1 large red pepper and 1 large yellow pepper, deseeded and cut into chunks

* 400g cauliflower, cut into small florets

* 1 tsp cumin seeds

Directions

* STEP 1

Heat the oven to 220C/200C fan/ gas 7. Boil the lentils for 35-40 mins over a medium heat until tender.

• STEP 2

Meanwhile, put the ginger, fresh coriander, garam masala, the ground coriander, ground cumin and the 2 whole garlic cloves in a large bowl with half the lemon juice and 3 tbsp of the yogurt. Blitz using a hand blender until smooth. Use 4 tbsp of the mixture to coat the chicken thighs in a large bowl. Arrange the chicken on a baking tray in a single layer.

• STEP 3

Add the remaining yogurt to the remaining spice and herb mixture, along with the turmeric, 1 tsp oil, the grated garlic, 1 tbsp water and remaining lemon juice to taste. Set aside.

• STEP 4

Tip the onions, peppers and cauliflower into the bowl used for the chicken, and toss with 1 tbsp oil to coat in some of the spice mix. Spread the veg out on a baking tray, then put in the oven with the chicken for 30-35 mins until the chicken is cooked through.

• STEP 5

Remove the chicken and wrap in foil to keep it warm. Scatter the cumin seeds over the veg and return to the oven for 5 mins until golden.

• STEP 6

To serve, drain the lentils and put in a serving bowl with the roasted veg and the remaining turmeric yogurt. Gently toss together. Serve with the chicken (taking the meat off the bones), and scatter with the extra coriander

Fennel, cherry & goat's cheese salad with lentils

Ingredients

• 50g walnut halves or pieces

• 250g pack pre-cooked puy lentils

• 1 large fennel bulb, finely sliced, fronds reserved

• 140g cherries, halved and pitted (or small figs, halved)

• 1 tbsp red wine vinegar

• 2 tbsp extra virgin olive oil

• 1 tsp Dijon mustard

• ½ tsp clear honey

• ½ small pack tarragon, roughly chopped

• 100g pack soft goat's cheese (any kind will work, but ash-rolled looks a bit special), thickly sliced and halved

Directions

• STEP 1

Heat a dry frying pan over a low-medium heat. Add the walnuts and cook for 3 mins, stirring frequently, until they smell toasty and the skins are a deep golden brown. Set aside to cool.

• STEP 2

Heat the lentils following pack instructions, then tip into a large bowl and loosen with a fork. Tip the fennel and cherries on top.

• STEP 3

Whisk together the vinegar, oil, mustard, honey and tarragon, then season. Fold the dressing through the lentils, fennel and cherries, then scoop the salad onto a platter. Scatter with the cheese, walnuts and the reserved fennel fronds.

Prosciutto, kale & butter bean stew

Ingredients

• 80g pack prosciutto, torn into pieces

• 2 tbsp olive oil

• 1 fennel bulb, sliced

• 2 garlic clove, crushed

• 1 tsp chilli flakes

• 4 thyme sprigs

• 150ml white wine or chicken stock

• 2 x 400g cans butter beans

• 400g can cherry tomatoes

• 200g bag sliced kale

Directions

• STEP 1

Fry the prosciutto in a dry saucepan over a high heat until crisp, then remove half with a slotted spoon and set aside. Turn the heat down to low, pour in the oil and tip in the fennel with a pinch of salt. Cook for 5 mins until softened, then throw in the garlic, chilli flakes and thyme and cook for a further 2 mins, then pour in the wine or stock and bring to a simmer.

• STEP 2

Tip both cans of butter beans into the stew, along with their liquid, then add the tomatoes, season well and bring everything to a simmer. Cook, undisturbed, for 5 mins, then stir through the kale. Once wilted, ladle the stew into bowls, removing the thyme sprigs and topping each portion with the remaining prosciutto.

Feta & kale loaded sweet potato

Ingredients

- 2 sweet potatoes

- chickpeas, drained

- 1 red onion, thinly sliced

- 2tbsp red wine vinegar

- 30g feta, cut into small cubes

- 1 tsp caster sugar

- 1tbsp olive oil

- chilli flakes

- 100g kale

• 1tbsp pumpkin seeds, toasted

• rocket

Directions

• STEP 1

Heat oven to 200C/180C fan/gas 6. Prick the sweet potatoes all over with a fork, then put them in a roasting tin and roast for 40 mins. Add the chickpeas to the tray, then roast for 10 mins more, until the potatoes are completely tender and the chickpeas have crisped a little.

• STEP 2

Meanwhile, mix the onion with the vinegar and a pinch of sugar and salt, and set aside to quick pickle. In another bowl, marinate the feta with the oil and chilli flakes.

• STEP 3

When the potatoes are nearly cooked, cook the kale in a pan with 50ml water for 3 mins until wilted, then season to taste. Halve the potatoes, divide between two plates and top each with the kale, chickpeas, red onion (reserving the vinegar), marinated feta and pumpkin seeds. Toss the rocket with the reserved vinegar, then serve on the side.

Kale & quinoa patties

Ingredients

• 140g quinoa

• 500g hot vegetable stock

- 100g kale, stalks removed, leaves roughly chopped

- 3 tbsp olive oil

- 1 small onion, finely chopped

- 2 garlic cloves, crushed

- 75g fresh white breadcrumbs

- 2 medium eggs, beaten

- 50g sundried tomatoes, roughly chopped

- 100g goat's cheese, cut from a round log

- green salad, to serve (optional)

For the pesto

- ½ small pack basil, leaves only

- ½ small pack parsley, leaves only

- 2 garlic cloves, crushed

- 50g pine nuts, toasted

- 50g parmesan, grated

- 150g olive oil

- juice 1 lemon

Directions

- STEP 1

Put the quinoa in a saucepan and pour over the hot stock. Simmer for 18-20 mins over a gentle heat until the grains have fluffed up and the liquid has disappeared. Remove from the heat and allow to cool. Meanwhile, bring a large saucepan of water to the boil. Add the kale and simmer for 6-8 mins until cooked through. Drain, squeeze out any excess water and set aside.

• STEP 2

Put 1 tbsp olive oil in a small frying pan over a medium heat. Add the onion and cook for 2-3 mins until translucent. Add the garlic and cook for 1 min more. Tip the cooked quinoa into a bowl and add the kale, onion, garlic, breadcrumbs, egg and sundried tomatoes. Season well and mix to combine. Set aside.

• STEP 3

To make the pesto, put the basil, parsley, garlic, pine nuts and Parmesan in a small food processor. Pulse, slowly pouring in the oil, until you have a thick pesto. Squeeze in the lemon juice to loosen, then set aside.

• STEP 4

Gently heat 2 tbsp olive oil in a shallow frying pan. Using your hands, form the quinoa mixture into 8 round patties. Add to the frying pan and fry for 4-5 mins each side until crisp and golden.

• STEP 5

Heat the grill to high and put a slice of goat's cheese on top of each patty. Place under the grill to brown and melt the cheese slightly – this will take a matter of seconds, so keep an eye on them. Top each patty with a generous spoonful of pesto and serve with some fresh green leaves, if you like.

Kale & chorizo broth

Ingredients

- 3 tbsp olive oil

- 2 onions, finely chopped

- 4 garlic cloves, crushed

- 2-3 cooking chorizo sausages, sliced

- 4 large potatoes

- 1 ½l chicken stock

- 200g curly kale, finely shredded

Directions

- STEP 1

Heat 2 tbsp of the oil in a large saucepan. Add the onions, garlic and chorizo, then cook for 5 mins until soft. Throw in the potatoes and cook for a few mins more. Pour in the stock, season and bring to the boil. Cook everything for 10 mins until the potatoes are on the brink of collapse.

• STEP 2

Use a masher to squash the potatoes into the soup, then bring back to the boil. Add the kale and cook for 5 mins until tender. Ladle the soup into bowls, then serve drizzled with the remaining olive oil.

Leek & butter bean soup with crispy kale & bacon

Ingredients

• 4 tsp olive oil

- 500g leeks, sliced

- 4 thyme sprigs, leaves picked

- 2 x 400g cans butter beans

- 500ml vegetable bouillon stock

- 2 tsp wholegrain mustard

- ½ small pack flat-leaf parsley

- 3 rashers streaky bacon

- 40g chopped kale, any tough stems removed

- 25g hazelnuts, roughly chopped

Directions

- STEP 1

Heat 1 tbsp oil in a large saucepan over a low heat. Add the leeks, thyme and seasoning. Cover and cook for 15 mins until softened, adding a splash of water if the leeks start to stick. Add the butter beans with the water from the cans, the stock and mustard. Bring to the boil and simmer for 3-4 mins until hot. Blend the soup in a food processor or with a stick blender, stir through the parsley and check the seasoning.

• STEP 2

Put the bacon in a large, non-stick frying pan over a medium heat. Cook for 3-4 mins until crispy, then set side to cool. Add the remaining 1 tsp oil to the pan, and tip in the kale and hazelnuts. Cook for 2 mins, stirring until the kale is wilted and crisping at the edges and the hazelnuts are toasted. Cut the bacon into small pieces, then stir into the kale mixture.

• STEP 3

Reheat the soup, adding a splash of water if it is too thick. Serve in bowls sprinkled with the bacon & kale mixture.

CHAPTER VII

NOURISHING DINNER RECIPES FOR LICHEN SCLEROSIS

Garlic prawns with puy lentils

Ingredients

• 400g raw, peeled tiger prawn, defrosted if frozen

• 2 red chillies, deseeded and finely chopped

• zest and juice 1 lime

• 2 large garlic cloves, crushed

• 2 tbsp oil

• 200g Puy lentil

For the dressing

• 2 tbsp soy sauce

• 1 tbsp clear honey

• 1 tbsp rice wine vinegar

• 3 tbsp sesame seed, toasted

• bunch coriander, leaves roughly chopped

Directions

• STEP 1

Place the prawns in a shallow dish. Mix together half the finely chopped chilli, lime zest and juice, garlic and oil, then pour over the prawns. Cover and chill for 20 mins to marinate.

• STEP 2

Meanwhile, put the lentils in a pan, cover with twice their depth in water, bring to the boil, then simmer for 15-20 mins until tender. Top up the water if you need to.

• STEP 3

To make the dressing, put the remaining chopped chilli, the soy, honey and vinegar into a small bowl and stir together. Drain the lentils, then tip into a large bowl. Spoon over almost all the dressing while the lentils are hot, tip in the sesame seeds, then mix well.

• STEP 4

Heat a frying pan until really hot. Lift the prawns out of the marinade, then fry for 1-2 mins each side until pink and lightly golden. Pour in the marinade and bring to the boil. Fold the chopped coriander through the lentils, then spoon onto serving plates. Top with the prawns and any pan juices.

Sticky sausage & sweet potato salad

Ingredients

• 8 pork sausages

• 600g sweet potato, cut into thin wedges

• 1 tbsp olive oil

• 2 tbsp wholegrain mustard

• 3 tbsp clear honey

• 200g bag baby spinach

For the dressing

• 5 tbsp olive oil

• 2 tbsp white wine vinegar

• 1 red onion, thinly sliced

Directions

• STEP 1

Heat oven to 200C/180C fan/gas 6. Toss the sausages and potatoes in a roasting tin with the oil. Roast for 30 mins, then mix the mustard and honey together and stir into the tin. Roast for 10 mins more until sticky and cooked.

• STEP 2

Meanwhile, mix together the dressing Ingredients with some seasoning – the onion will soften slightly in the vinegar.

• STEP 3

When the sausages are ready, thickly slice them, then mix back in with the potatoes. Tip the spinach onto plates, pile the sticky sausage slices and potatoes on top, then spoon over the dressing.

Open leek & sweet potato pie

Ingredients

• 3 tbsp olive oil, plus extra for brushing

• 2 large leeks, washed and sliced

• 2 sweet potatoes, peeled and roughly chopped into 2cm cubes

• 1 tsp coriander seeds

• 1 tsp chilli flakes

• 2 fat garlic cloves, crushed

• 150g ricotta

• 2 large eggs

• 1 lemon, zested

• 100g robust leafy greens such as cavalo nero or kale, finely shredded, tough core removed

• 1 small pack dill, chopped

• 1 pack filo pastry (around 12 sheets)

• 80g goat's cheese

• 1 tsp nigella seeds (optional)

• peppery salad, to serve

Directions

• STEP 1

Heat the oil in a large ovenproof frying pan. Add the leeks and a pinch of salt, then cook over a medium heat for a couple of mins until beginning to wilt. Tip in the sweet potato, cover the pan then cook, stirring occasionally, for 15 mins until the potato is mostly softened. Stir in the coriander seeds, chilli flakes, garlic and season. Give everything a gentle stir – you want the potato to remain intact as much as possible – then remove the pan from the heat and set aside to cool slightly.

• STEP 2

In a large bowl, whisk together the ricotta, eggs and lemon zest with some seasoning. Stir in the greens and dill, then scrape in the sweet potato filling, (set aside the frying pan afterwards) and fold everything together. Heat oven to 220C/200C fan/gas 7.

• STEP 3

Lay your first sheet of filo in the frying pan you used for the sweet potato (no need to wash it first). Brush the top with a little oil, then continue to layer the filo, setting each sheet at a different angle and oiling in between the layers until all edges of the pan are covered. Spoon the filling on top of the pastry, dot over the goat's cheese, then crumple the pastry in over the filling, leaving the centre of the pie exposed. Brush the top with a little more oil and scatter over the nigella seeds, if using.

• STEP 4

Turn the hob back on and cook the pie over a medium-low heat for 3 mins to ensure the base is crisp, then transfer to the oven and bake for 12-15 mins until the pastry is crisp and golden. Let the pie cool in the pan for 10 mins before slicing.

Homemade burgers with sweet potato wedges

Ingredients

For the burgers

• 1 tbsp olive oil, plus extra for drizzling

• 1 red onion, finely chopped

• 500g lean minced beef or turkey

- 1 egg

- 12 cream crackers, bashed to fine crumbs

- 2 tsp chilli paste

- 2 tsp garlic paste

- 1 tsp each, tomato ketchup and brown sauce

- 2 tbsp plain flour

- 6 hamburger rolls, toasted, to serve

- toppings of your choice (relish, chutney and salad), to serve

For the wedges

- 4 sweet potatoes, cut into wedges

• 2 tbsp olive oil

• 1 tsp paprika

Directions

• STEP 1

Heat the oil in a frying pan and fry the onion for about 5 mins or until soft. Leave to cool slightly. When cool, put the onion in a large bowl with the mince, egg, bashed crackers, chilli, garlic, ketchup and brown sauce, and mix well to combine. Divide the mince into 6, roll into balls and flatten each into a nice fat burger.

• STEP 2

Put the flour on a plate, dab each burger to the flour on both sides, then transfer to a baking tray. Wrap with cling film and pop in the fridge for a couple of hours.

• STEP 3

Heat oven to 200C/180C fan/gas 6. To make the wedges, put the sweet potato on a baking tray and drizzle with olive oil. Sprinkle with paprika, season, then give them a good shake or shuffle around with your hands to make sure they're well coated. Roast for 30-40 mins depending on how crisp you like them. Make sure you give them a good shake a couple of times to ensure they cook evenly.

• STEP 4

When the wedges have been cooking for 10 mins, drizzle the burgers with a little olive oil and put them in the oven to cook with the wedges for the remaining 20-30 mins, flipping them halfway. 5

Serve the burgers in the rolls with your choice of toppings, and a good helping of wedges on the side.

Spicy turkey sweet potatoes

Ingredients

• 4 sweet potatoes

• 1 tbsp olive oil

• 1 onion, finely chopped

• 1 garlic clove, crushed

• 500g pack turkey thigh mince

• 500g carton passata

• 3 tbsp barbecue sauce

• ½ tsp cayenne pepper

• 4 tbsp soured cream

• ½ pack chives, finely snipped

Directions

• STEP 1

Heat oven to 200C/180C fan/gas 6. Prick the potatoes, place on a baking tray and bake for 45 mins or until really soft.

• STEP 2

Meanwhile, heat the oil in a frying pan, add the onion and cook gently for 8 mins until softened. Stir in the garlic, then tip in the mince and stir to break up. Cook over a high heat until any liquid has evaporated and the mince is browned, about 10 mins. Pour in the passata, then fill the carton a quarter full of water and tip that in too. Add the barbecue sauce and cayenne, then lower the heat and simmer gently for 15 mins, adding a little extra water if needed. Taste and season.

• STEP 3

When the potatoes are soft, split them down the centre and spoon the mince over the top. Add a dollop of soured cream and a sprinkling of chives

Roast squash with goat's cheese & puy lentils

Ingredients

• 800g delicata, acorn or butternut squash

• 4 tbsp rapeseed or olive oil

• 25g pumpkin seeds (or use the seeds from the pumpkin or squash you're using)

• 10 sage leaves

• 2 tbsp good-quality red wine vinegar

• 250g pouch cooked puy lentils

• 100g soft goat's cheese

• 4 amaretti biscuits

For the crispy kale

• 100g kale, rinsed, dried, thick stems removed and leaves torn into crisp-sized pieces

• ½ tbsp rapeseed or olive oil

• 1 tbsp white sesame seeds

• 1 tsp red chilli flakes

Procedure

• STEP 1

Heat oven to 160C/140C fan/gas 3. Toss the kale lightly in the oil, ½ tsp salt, sesame and chilli, massaging the leaves until coated with the oil and seasoning. Arrange the leaves in one layer in a roasting tin or baking tray – you might need to use more than one to keep them in an even layer. Roast for 15-20 mins until crisp and dry but not brown.

• STEP 2

Once dried, remove from the oven and turn the heat up to 200C/180C fan/gas 6. Halve the squash and scoop out the seeds. Wash the seeds to remove the sticky membrane, dry them with kitchen paper and set aside. Cut the squash into 1cm thick slices (don't worry about peeling them), and arrange on a baking sheet or in a roasting tin. Drizzle over 1 tbsp oil, season, then turn and drizzle with a little more oil. Season again and roast for 30-40 mins until tender and caramelising, turning halfway through. Remove from the oven.

• STEP 3

Heat the remaining oil in a non-stick frying pan over a medium to high heat until it's shimmering. Add the sage leaves and fry for 15-30 seconds, turning them once. Remove using tongs or a slotted spoon, place on kitchen paper and scatter with sea salt. Add the pumpkin seeds to the hot oil and fry for a few mins until puffed and crunchy. Drain the oil into a bowl and whisk with the red wine vinegar, a pinch of salt and freshly ground black pepper.

• STEP 4

Dress the lentils with half the dressing, then spoon onto the plates or serving platter. Arrange the crispy kale and squash on top, crumble over the goat's cheese, and drizzle over a bit more dressing. Finally, top with the fried seeds, and crumble over the amaretti biscuits and crispy sage leaves.

Chipolatas in apple gravy with parsnip colcannon

Ingredients

• 1 large potato, cut into chunks

• 4 parsnips, peeled and cut into chunks

• 8 chipolatas

* 50g butter

* 2 large red apples, cored and cut into slim wedges

* 8 spring onions, sliced, white and green parts separated

* 1 tbsp flour

* 1 beef or chicken stock cube

* 200g kale or Savoy cabbage, finely chopped

* 5ml milk

Procedure

* STEP 1

Put the potato and parsnips in a very large pan of water, bring to the boil and simmer for 10 mins or until the veg is tender. Meanwhile, cook the chipolatas in a large frying pan. When brown on all sides, transfer to a plate and add 25g butter to the pan. Add the apples and white part of the spring onions. Fry for 5-10 mins until softened and starting to caramelise.

• STEP 2

Add the kale to the boiling veg for the final few mins, before the potatoes and parsnips are completely soft. When the kale has wilted, drain the veg and leave to steam-dry in the colander. Heat the remaining butter in the same pan – don't worry about washing it out. Add the green parts of the spring onions and sizzle for a few mins to soften.

• STEP 3

Add the flour and stock cube to the apples and spring onions, stir for 1-2 mins, then add 400ml water, mixing to a smooth gravy. Return the sausages to the pan and bubble in the gravy for a few mins until heated through. Meanwhile, add the veg to the buttery spring onions, along with the milk and plenty of seasoning, and mash until the potato and parsnips are smooth. Serve the colcannon with the chipolatas and the gravy spooned over the top.

Salsa verde salmon with smashed chickpea salad

Ingredients

• 3 tsp olive oil

• 1 orange, zested and juiced

• 2 skin-on salmon fillets

• small bunch of parsley (including stalks), finely chopped

• ½ tbsp Dijon mustard

• 1 shallot or 1/2 small red onion, finely chopped

• ½ tbsp red wine vinegar

• 400g can chickpeas, drained and rinsed

• 2 roasted red peppers from a jar, drained and chopped

• 50g kale

Procedure

• STEP 1

Heat the grill to high. Whisk 1 tsp of the oil with the orange zest, a splash of the juice, lots of black pepper and a small pinch of salt. Put the salmon, skin-side down, on a non-stick baking tray and pour over the marinade. Leave to marinate at room temperature while you make the salsa.

• STEP 2

Put the parsley, mustard, half the shallot, the vinegar, 1 tsp oil, and the remaining orange juice in a small food processor and blitz to a thick sauce, adding a splash of water to loosen if needed.

• STEP 3

Heat the remaining oil in a frying pan and fry the remaining shallot for 5 mins. Stir in the chickpeas and some seasoning, turn up the heat and stir until the chickpeas are just starting to crisp. Mash roughly with a potato masher and stir in the roasted peppers and kale. Add a splash of water and cover with a lid until the kale is wilted. Keep warm over a low heat.

• STEP 4

Grill the salmon for 4-6 mins, or until cooked to your liking. Spoon half the chickpeas onto a plate, top with a salmon fillet (leaving the skin behind if you like), and spoon over some of the salsa verde. Leave the remaining salmon fillet to cool to use in the lunchbox, see tip below.

RECIPE TIPS

FOR THE LEFTOVER LUNCHBOX

Put the leftover chickpea salad into a lunchbox with some halved cherry tomatoes. Flake over the leftover salmon, and top with the remaining salsa verde. Chill overnight, or until ready to eat.

Veggie tahini lentils

Ingredients

• 50g tahini

• zest and juice 1 lemon

• 2 tbsp olive oil

• 1 red onion, thinly sliced

• 1 garlic clove, crushed

• 1 yellow pepper, thinly sliced

• 200g green beans, trimmed and halved

- 1 courgette, sliced into half moons

- 100g shredded kale

- 250g pack pre-cooked puy lentils

Procedure

- STEP 1

In a jug, mix the tahini with the zest and juice of the lemon and 50ml of cold water to make a runny dressing. Season to taste, then set aside.

- STEP 2

Heat the oil in a wok or large frying pan over a medium-high heat. Add the red onion, along with a pinch of salt, and fry for 2 mins until starting to soften and colour. Add the garlic, pepper, green beans and courgette and fry for 5 min, stirring frequently.

• STEP 3

Tip in the kale, lentils and the tahini dressing. Keep the pan on the heat for a couple of mins, stirring everything together until the kale is wilted and it's all coated in the creamy dressing.

Kale & apple soup with walnuts

Ingredients

• 8 walnut halves, broken into pieces

• 1 onion, finely chopped

• 2 carrots, coarsely grated

* 2 red apples, unpeeled and finely chopped

* 1 tbsp cider vinegar

* 500ml reduced-salt vegetable stock

* 200g kale, roughly chopped

* 20g pack of dried apple crisps (optional)

Procedure

* STEP 1

In a dry, non-stick frying pan, cook the walnut pieces for 2-3 mins until toasted, turning frequently so they don't burn. Take off the heat and allow to cool.

* STEP 2

Put the onion, carrots, apples, vinegar and stock in a large saucepan and bring to the boil. Reduce the heat and simmer for 10 mins, stirring occasionally.

• STEP 3

Once the onion is translucent and the apples start to soften, add the kale and simmer for an additional 2 mins. Carefully transfer to a blender or liquidiser and blend until very smooth. Pour into bowls and serve topped with the toasted walnuts, and a sprinkling of apple crisps, if you like.

Sausage, kale & gnocchi one-pot

Ingredients

• 1 tbsp olive oil

• 6 pork sausages

- 1 tsp chilli flakes

- 1 tsp fennel seeds (optional)

- 500g fresh gnocchi

- 500ml chicken stock (fresh if you can get it)

- 100g chopped kale

- 40g parmesan, finely grated

Directions

- STEP 1

Heat the oil in a large high-sided frying pan over a medium heat. Squeeze the sausages straight from their skins into the pan, then use the back of a wooden spoon to break the meat up. Sprinkle in the chilli flakes and fennel seeds, if using, then fry until the sausagemeat is crisp around the edges. Remove from the pan with a slotted spoon.

• STEP 2

Tip the gnocchi into the pan, fry for a minute or so, then pour in the chicken stock. Once bubbling, cover the pan with a lid and cook for 3 mins, then stir in the kale. Cook for 2 mins more or until the gnocchi is tender and the kale has wilted. Stir in the parmesan, then season with black pepper and scatter the crisp sausagemeat over the top.

Spiced black bean & chicken soup with kale

Ingredients

• 2 tbsp mild olive oil

- 2 fat garlic cloves, crushed

- small bunch coriander stalks finely chopped, leaves picked

- zest 1 lime, then cut into wedges

- 2 tsp ground cumin

- 1 tsp chilli flakes

- 400g can chopped tomatoes

- 400g can black beans, rinsed and drained

- 600ml chicken stock

- 175g kale, thick stalks removed, leaves shredded

- 250g leftover roast or ready-cooked chicken

* 50g feta, crumbled, to serve

* flour & corn tortillas, toasted, to serve

Directions

* STEP 1

Heat the oil in a large saucepan, add the garlic, coriander stalks and lime zest, then fry for 2 mins until fragrant. Stir in the cumin and chilli flakes, fry for 1 min more, then tip in the tomatoes, beans and stock. Bring to the boil, then crush the beans against the bottom of the pan a few times using a potato masher. This will thicken the soup a little.

* STEP 2

Stir the kale into the soup, simmer for 5 mins or until tender, then tear in the chicken and let it heat through. Season to taste with salt, pepper and juice from half the lime, then serve in shallow bowls, scattered with the feta and a few coriander leaves. Serve the remaining lime in wedges for the table, with the toasted tortillas on the side. The longer you leave the chicken in the pan, the thicker the soup will become, so add a splash more stock if you can't serve the soup straight away.

Creamy pesto & kale pasta

Ingredients

- 1 tbsp rapeseed oil

- 2 red onions, thinly sliced

- 300g kale

• 300g wholemeal pasta (penne or mafalda work well)

• 4 tbsp reduced-fat soft cheese

• 4 tbsp fresh or jar pesto, or vegetarian alternative

Directions

• STEP 1

Heat the oil in a large pan over a medium heat. Fry the onions for 10 mins until softened and beginning to caramelise. Add the kale and 100ml water, then cover and cook for 5 mins more, or until the kale has wilted.

• STEP 2

Cook the pasta following pack instructions. Drain, reserving a little of the cooking water. Toss the pasta with the onion mixture, soft cheese and pesto, adding a splash of the reserved cooking water to loosen, if needed. Season.

Coconut & kale fish curry

Ingredients

• 1 tbsp rapeseed oil

• 1 onion, sliced

• thumb-sized piece ginger, sliced into matchsticks

• 1 tsp turmeric

• 3-4 tbsp mild curry paste (Keralan works well)

• 150g cherry tomatoes, halved

• 150g kale, chopped

• 1 red chilli, halved

• 325ml reduced fat coconut milk

• 300ml low-salt stock

• 250g brown rice

• 100g frozen king prawns

• 2 cod fillets, cut into chunks

• 2 limes, juiced

• ½ small bunch coriander, chopped

• handful of toasted coconut flakes (optional)

Directions

• STEP 1

Heat the oil in a casserole dish. Cook the onion with a pinch of salt for 10 mins until it starts to caramalise. Stir through the ginger, turmeric and curry paste, and cook for 2 mins.

• STEP 2

Add the tomatoes, kale and chilli, and pour in the coconut milk and stock. Simmer for 10-15 mins or until the tomatoes begin to soften. Scoop out the chilli and discard.

• STEP 3

Cook the rice following pack instructions. Gently stir the prawns and cod through the curry, then cook for another 3-5 mins. Squeeze over the lime and stir through half of the coriander. To serve, scatter over the remaining coriander and the coconut flakes, if you like. Serve with the rice.

Sausage & kale minestrone

Ingredients

• 1 tbsp vegetable oil

• 1 red onion, finely chopped

• 3 sausages, skins removed

• 2 garlic cloves, finely grated

• ½-1 red chilli, depending on how much heat you prefer, sliced

• ½ large head of broccoli, finely chopped

• 2 courgettes, sliced into half-moons

• 200g small pasta (we used ditalini)

• 1½ litres chicken stock, made with low-salt chicken stock cube

• 200g curly kale or cavolo nero, stalks removed, roughly chopped

• 1 lemon, zested and juiced

• 20g parmesan, shaved

Directions

• STEP 1

Heat the oil over a medium heat in a large, deep pot that has a lid. Cook the onion for 10 mins until softened and golden at the edges.

• STEP 2

Crumble in the sausages, breaking them into bite-sized pieces using a spoon. Cook for 7-8 mins until golden and crisp. Stir in the garlic and chilli.

• STEP 3

Add the broccoli and courgettes. Cook for 10-12 mins until soft, then pour in the pasta and chicken stock. Stir to combine, then bring to a boil. Reduce to a simmer, put the lid on and cook for 8-10 mins, until the pasta is almost cooked.

• STEP 4

Wilt in the kale or cavolo nero in batches and cook for a further 2-3 mins, until the kale is cooked and the pasta is al dente. Squeeze in the lemon juice and season well. Divide between four bowls and sprinkle over the lemon zest and parmesan shavings to serve.

CHAPTER VIII

NOURISHING MAIN COURSE RECIPES FOR LICHEN SCLEROSIS

One-pot chicken with chorizo & new potatoes

Ingredients

• 1 whole chicken (about 1.5kg), the best quality you can afford

• small knob of butter

• 1 tbsp olive oil

• ½ lemon

• 1 bay leaf

• 1 thyme sprig

• 300g chorizo ring, thickly sliced

• 700g new potatoes, halved (or quartered if really large)

• 12 garlic cloves, left whole and unpeeled

• large splash of dry sherry

• 150ml chicken stock

• handful parsley leaves, roughly chopped

Directions

• STEP 1

Heat oven to 180C/160C fan/gas 4 and season the chicken all over. In a large flameproof casserole dish with a lid, heat the butter and oil until sizzling, then spend a good 15 mins slowly browning the chicken well all over. Remove from the dish and pop the lemon, bay and thyme in the cavity. Set aside.

• STEP 2

Pour most of the oil out of the dish, place back on the heat and sizzle the chorizo for 5 mins until it starts to release its red oil. Throw in the potatoes, sizzle them until they start to colour, then add the garlic. Splash in the sherry, let it bubble down a little, then pour in the stock.

• STEP 3

Nestle the chicken, breast-side up, among the potatoes, place the lid on the dish and cook in the oven for 1 hr 15 mins or until the legs easily come away from the body. Leave the chicken to rest for 10 mins, then scatter with parsley and serve straight from the dish.

Domino potato, cod, prawn & chorizo pie

Ingredients

• 850g floury potatoes, such as Maris Piper

• 500g cod fillet, skin and pin bones removed

• 650ml full-fat milk

• 6 bay leaves

• good pinch of saffron

• 1 tbsp olive oil, plus a drizzle

- 50g butter

- 1 large onion, halved and finely sliced

- 1 fennel, quartered and finely sliced

- 2 garlic cloves, crushed

- 200g chorizo ring, skin removed and sliced

- 50g plain flour

- small bunch parsley, chopped

- 200g king prawns, peeled

- green salad or veg, to serve

Directions

- STEP 1

Peel and thinly slice the potatoes, tip into a pan of cold water and bring to a simmer. Turn off the heat, leave the potatoes in the water for 1 min, then drain and leave to cool in a colander. The potatoes should still feel firm and hold their shape. Put the cod in a wide, deep pan and pour over the milk. Add 2 bay leaves and saffron and bring to a gentle simmer, cover with a lid, then lower the heat and cook for 2 mins. Turn off the heat and leave the fish in the pan to continue cooking for 5 mins more.

• STEP 2

Heat the oil and butter in another large pan, add the onion and fennel and cook for 10 mins until starting to caramelise. Add the garlic and chorizo, stir until the oils are released, then stir in the flour.

• STEP 3

Remove the fish from the milk and set aside the bay leaves. Add the milk to the chorizo pan bit by bit, stirring between additions, until you have a smooth, thick sauce. Stir in the parsley, season and remove from the heat.

• STEP 4

Heat oven to 200C/180C fan/gas 6. Pour half of the sauce into a large casserole dish. Flake the fish into large chunks and scatter over the sauce. Add the prawns and spoon over the rest of the sauce.

• STEP 5

Stack 5-6 potato slices together and trim off the edges to create a rectangle– don't worry if it's not perfect. Continue making stacks of rectangular potatoes until they're all used up. Scatter the trimmings over the sauce, then arrange the slices on top in a domino pattern, fanning them out to cover the surface. Tuck the reserved bay leaves and four others in among the potatoes, season and drizzle with oil. Bake for 45 mins until the potatoes are tender and golden and the sauce is bubbling up around the edges. Serve with green veg or salad.

Warm new potato salad with bacon & blue cheese

Ingredients

• 500g salad potato, halved

• 2 tbsp olive oil

• 2 red onions, each sliced into 6 wedges

• 4 rashers smoked back bacon, trimmed and cut into large pieces

• 140g mushroom, sliced

• 1 tbsp wholegrain mustard

• 1 tbsp red wine vinegar

• 100g bag mixed watercress and spinach salad

• 85g creamy blue cheese (we used St Agur)

Directions

• STEP 1

Heat oven to 220C/fan 200C/gas 7. Place the potatoes in a roasting tin, then rub with 1 tbsp oil and a sprinkling of salt. Roast for 20 mins, then add the onion wedges to the tin, giving everything a good shake. Roast for 20 mins more until the potatoes have turned a deep golden brown and the onions have caramelised and softened. Leave to cool slightly.

• STEP 2

Heat a non-stick frying pan. Dry-fry the bacon until crisp. Add the sliced mushrooms, then fry for 5 mins more until they have softened.

• STEP 3

Meanwhile, make the dressing. Whisk the mustard, vinegar and remaining 1 tbsp oil with a splash of water. Place potatoes, onions, bacon and mushrooms in a large bowl with the salad leaves, pour over the dressing, then toss well. Divide between 4 plates, then crumble over the blue cheese.

Warm new potato & smoked mackerel salad

Ingredients

• 350g new potato

• 100g crème fraîche

• 1 tsp horseradish cream

• juice of 1 lemon

• 2 smoked mackerel fillets (about 200g/8oz total weight), skinned and flaked

• 85g bag watercress

Directions

• STEP 1

Cook the potatoes in a large pan of boiling salted water for 15-20 minutes or until tender.

• STEP 2

While the potatoes are cooking, mix the crème fraîche in a large bowl with the horseradish cream and lemon juice. Season well with freshly ground black pepper (there's no need for salt because of the saltiness of the smoked mackerel).

• STEP 3

Drain the potatoes, halve and set aside to cool down for a few minutes. Tip into the crème fraîche mix and stir so it coats them and becomes quite runny. Now add the smoked mackerel and watercress and toss gently together. Pile on two plates and serve straight away (it's best while still warm).

Curried chicken & new potato traybake

Ingredients

• 8 chicken drumsticks

• 3 tbsp olive oil

• 1 tsp garlic paste

• 1 tsp ginger paste

• 1 tsp garam masala

• 1 tsp turmeric

• 150ml pot natural yogurt

- 500g new potatoes, halved

- 4 large tomatoes, roughly chopped

- 1 red onion, finely chopped

- small pack coriander, roughly chopped

Directions

- STEP 1

Put the drumsticks in a large bowl with 1 tbsp oil, the garlic, ginger, garam masala, turmeric and 2 tbsp yogurt. Toss together with your hands until coated. Leave to marinate for at least 30 mins (can be left in the fridge overnight). Heat oven to 180C/160C fan/gas 4.

- STEP 2

Put the potatoes in a large roasting tin with the remaining oil and plenty of seasoning. Add the chicken drumsticks and bake for 40-45 mins until cooked and golden.

• STEP 3

Scatter the tomatoes, onion, coriander and some seasoning over the chicken and potatoes, with the remaining yogurt served on the side.

Vegan chickpea curry jacket potatoes

Ingredients

• 4 sweet potatoes

• 1 tbsp coconut oil

• 1 ½ tsp cumin seeds

- 1 large onion, diced

- 2 garlic cloves, crushed

- thumb-sized piece ginger, finely grated

- 1 green chilli, finely chopped

- 1 tsp garam masala

- 1 tsp ground coriander

- ½ tsp turmeric

- 2 tbsp tikka masala paste

- 2 x 400g can chopped tomatoes

- 2 x 400g can chickpeas, drained

- lemon wedges and coriander leaves, to serve

Directions

• STEP 1

Heat oven to 200C/180C fan/gas 6. Prick the sweet potatoes all over with a fork, then put on a baking tray and roast in the oven for 45 mins or until tender when pierced with a knife.

• STEP 2

Meanwhile, melt the coconut oil in a large saucepan over medium heat. Add the cumin seeds and fry for 1 min until fragrant, then add the onion and fry for 7-10 mins until softened.

• STEP 3

Put the garlic, ginger and green chilli into the pan, and cook for 2-3 mins. Add the spices and tikka masala paste and cook for a further 2 mins until fragrant, then tip in the tomatoes. Bring to a simmer, then tip in the chickpeas and cook for a further 20 mins until thickened. Season.

• STEP 4

Put the roasted sweet potatoes on four plates and cut open lengthways. Spoon over the chickpea curry and squeeze over the lemon wedges. Season, then scatter with coriander before serving.

Miso chilli steak with crispy sweet potatoes

Ingredients

• 2 large sweet potatoes, cut into wedges

• 1 tbsp vegetable oil, plus a little extra

* 1 tbsp sesame seed

* 1 tbsp miso paste

* juice 1 lemon

* 1 tbsp hot chilli sauce (sriracha is nice)

* 1 tbsp mirin

* 2 bavette or other lean steaks (about 200g each)

* large handful watercress leaves, to serve

Directions

* STEP 1

Heat oven to 200C/180C fan/gas 6. Put the potato wedges on a baking tray and rub with the oil.

Sprinkle the sesame seeds and some seasoning over. Bake for 25 mins or until crisp at the edges.

• STEP 2

In a small bowl, mix together the miso, lemon juice, chilli sauce and mirin. Rub the steaks with a tiny bit of oil and some seasoning. Spoon 1 tbsp of the sauce over each steak and rub into both sides.

• STEP 3

Heat a griddle pan until really hot, cook the steaks for 2 mins each side, or longer if you prefer it well done. Brush more of the sauce over after you turn them. Transfer to a plate, cover loosely with foil, and leave to rest for 5 mins. Serve the steaks sliced, with extra sauce, the potatoes and watercress.

Sausage, kale & gnocchi one-pot

Ingredients

- 1 tbsp olive oil

- 6 pork sausages

- 1 tsp chilli flakes

- 1 tsp fennel seeds (optional)

- 500g fresh gnocchi

- 500ml chicken stock (fresh if you can get it)

- 100g chopped kale

- 40g parmesan, finely grated

Directions

• STEP 1

Heat the oil in a large high-sided frying pan over a medium heat. Squeeze the sausages straight from their skins into the pan, then use the back of a wooden spoon to break the meat up. Sprinkle in the chilli flakes and fennel seeds, if using, then fry until the sausagemeat is crisp around the edges. Remove from the pan with a slotted spoon.

• STEP 2

Tip the gnocchi into the pan, fry for a minute or so, then pour in the chicken stock. Once bubbling, cover the pan with a lid and cook for 3 mins, then stir in the kale. Cook for 2 mins more or until the gnocchi is tender and the kale has wilted. Stir in the parmesan, then season with black pepper and scatter the crisp sausagemeat over the top.

Red lentil, chickpea & chilli soup

Ingredients

• 2 tsp cumin seeds

• large pinch chilli flakes

• 1 tbsp olive oil

• 1 red onion, chopped

• 140g red split lentils

• 850ml vegetable stock or water

• 400g can tomatoes, whole or chopped

• 200g can chickpeas or ½ a can, drained and rinsed (freeze leftovers)

• small bunch coriander, roughly chopped (save a few leaves, to serve)

• 4 tbsp 0% Greek yogurt, to serve

Directions

• STEP 1

Heat a large saucepan and dry-fry 2 tsp cumin seeds and a large pinch of chilli flakes for 1 min, or until they start to jump around the pan and release their aromas.

• STEP 2

Add 1 tbsp olive oil and 1 chopped red onion, and cook for 5 mins.

• STEP 3

Stir in 140g red split lentils, 850ml vegetable stock or water and a 400g can tomatoes, then bring to the boil. Simmer for 15 mins until the lentils have softened.

• STEP 4

Whizz the soup with a stick blender or in a food processor until it is a rough purée, pour back into the pan and add a 200g can drained and rinsed chickpeas.

• STEP 5

Heat gently, season well and stir in a small bunch of chopped coriander, reserving a few leaves to serve. Finish with 4 tbsp 0% Greek yogurt and extra coriander leaves.

Coconut & kale fish curry

Ingredients

• 1 tbsp rapeseed oil

• 1 onion, sliced

• thumb-sized piece ginger, sliced into matchsticks

• 1 tsp turmeric

• 3-4 tbsp mild curry paste (Keralan works well)

• 150g cherry tomatoes, halved

• 150g kale, chopped

• 1 red chilli, halved

• 325ml reduced fat coconut milk

• 300ml low-salt stock

• 250g brown rice

• 100g frozen king prawns

• 2 cod fillets, cut into chunks

• 2 limes, juiced

• ½ small bunch coriander, chopped

• handful of toasted coconut flakes (optional)

Directions

• STEP 1

Heat the oil in a casserole dish. Cook the onion with a pinch of salt for 10 mins until it starts to caramalise. Stir through the ginger, turmeric and curry paste, and cook for 2 mins.

• STEP 2

Add the tomatoes, kale and chilli, and pour in the coconut milk and stock. Simmer for 10-15 mins or until the tomatoes begin to soften. Scoop out the chilli and discard.

• STEP 3

Cook the rice following pack instructions. Gently stir the prawns and cod through the curry, then cook for another 3-5 mins. Squeeze over the lime and stir through half of the coriander. To serve, scatter over the remaining coriander and the coconut flakes, if you like. Serve with the rice.

Veggie tahini lentils

Ingredients

• 50g tahini

• zest and juice 1 lemon

• 2 tbsp olive oil

• 1 red onion, thinly sliced

• 1 garlic clove, crushed

• 1 yellow pepper, thinly sliced

• 200g green beans, trimmed and halved

• 1 courgette, sliced into half moons

• 100g shredded kale

• 250g pack pre-cooked puy lentils

Directions

• STEP 1

In a jug, mix the tahini with the zest and juice of the lemon and 50ml of cold water to make a runny dressing. Season to taste, then set aside.

• STEP 2

Heat the oil in a wok or large frying pan over a medium-high heat. Add the red onion, along with a pinch of salt, and fry for 2 mins until starting to soften and colour. Add the garlic, pepper, green beans and courgette and fry for 5 min, stirring frequently.

• STEP 3

Tip in the kale, lentils and the tahini dressing. Keep the pan on the heat for a couple of mins, stirring everything together until the kale is wilted and it's all coated in the creamy dressing.

Kale with chana & coconut

Ingredients

• 1 tbsp butter

• 1 onion, finely chopped

• thumb-sized piece ginger, grated

• 2 heaped tsp cumin seeds

• 1 tsp turmeric

• 1 tsp ground coriander

• 2 tbsp tomato purée

• 200g kale, large stalks removed, leaves finely shredded

• 400g can chickpeas, drained

• 250ml vegetable stock

• 50g fresh coconut, grated

• 4 heaped tbsp Greek-style yogurt

• 1 tbsp mango chutney

To serve

• 1 tbsp vegetable oil

• 3 garlic cloves, thinly sliced

• 2 tbsp freeze-dried curry leaves (optional)

Directions

• STEP 1

Heat the butter in a deep frying pan, add the onion, then soften gently for 5 mins. Turn up the heat and add the ginger and spices; fry for 2 mins until fragrant. Stir in the tomato purée.

• STEP 2

Add the kale, chickpeas, stock and two-thirds of the coconut, stir well, then cover the pan. Bring to a simmer and let the kale steam for 10 mins until very well wilted. Mix in the yogurt and chutney, then season to taste - don't boil once the yogurt has gone in. Remove the pan from the heat, and leave it covered to stay warm.

• STEP 3

Heat the oil in a small saucepan. When it's hot, add the garlic (and curry leaves, if using) and sizzle for 30 secs-1 min until the garlic begins to turn golden. Spoon the oil, garlic and curry leaves over the chickpeas and kale, then finish with the remaining coconut.

Prosciutto, kale & butter bean stew

Ingredients

• 80g pack prosciutto, torn into pieces

• 2 tbsp olive oil

• 1 fennel bulb, sliced

• 2 garlic clove, crushed

• 1 tsp chilli flakes

• 4 thyme sprigs

• 150ml white wine or chicken stock

• 2 x 400g cans butter beans

• 400g can cherry tomatoes

• 200g bag sliced kale

Directions

• STEP 1

Fry the prosciutto in a dry saucepan over a high heat until crisp, then remove half with a slotted spoon and set aside. Turn the heat down to low, pour in the oil and tip in the fennel with a pinch of salt. Cook for 5 mins until softened, then throw in the garlic, chilli flakes and thyme and cook for a further 2 mins, then pour in the wine or stock and bring to a simmer.

• STEP 2

Tip both cans of butter beans into the stew, along with their liquid, then add the tomatoes, season well and bring everything to a simmer. Cook, undisturbed, for 5 mins, then stir through the kale. Once wilted, ladle the stew into bowls, removing the thyme sprigs and topping each portion with the remaining prosciutto.

Kale pesto

Ingredients

• 85g pine nut, toasted

• 85g parmesan (or vegetarian alternative), coarsely grated, plus extra to serve (optional)

• 3 garlic cloves

• 75ml extra-virgin olive oil, plus extra to serve

• 75ml olive oil

• 85g kale

• juice 1 lemon

• spaghetti or linguine, to serve

Directions

• STEP 1

Put the pine nuts, Parmesan, garlic, oils, kale and lemon juice in a food processor and whizz to a paste. Season to taste. Stir through hot pasta to serve, topping with extra Parmesan and olive oil, if you like.

• STEP 2

To store, put in a container or jar, cover the surface with a little more olive oil and keep in the fridge for a week, or freeze for up to a month.

CHAPTER IX

BEFORE YOU LEAVE, A FINAL WORD!

There is no single diet for lichen sclerosis; however, consuming foods that are low in oxalate can potentially reduce the symptoms associated with the disease. Consuming foods that are high in oxalate can aggravate the inflammation.

Certain irritants such as shower gels, bubble baths, and detergents can worsen itchiness and lead to skin tears. In addition, avoid wearing restrictive or tight underwear; instead, wear the types made of silk or cotton. Other tips to alleviate lichen sclerosis include staying hydrated and consuming foods that contain healthy fats.

Regardless, it is important to consult a licensed health professional immediately if you notice any abnormality on the skin, especially around or on the genitals. You can consult a dietitian to get appropriate and customized recommendations for a low-oxalate diet or other available options.

www.ingramcontent.com/pod-product-compliance
Lightning Source LLC
Chambersburg PA
CBHW061037250726
48653CB00001B/137